Everything
You Need to
Know About

Multiple
Sclerosis

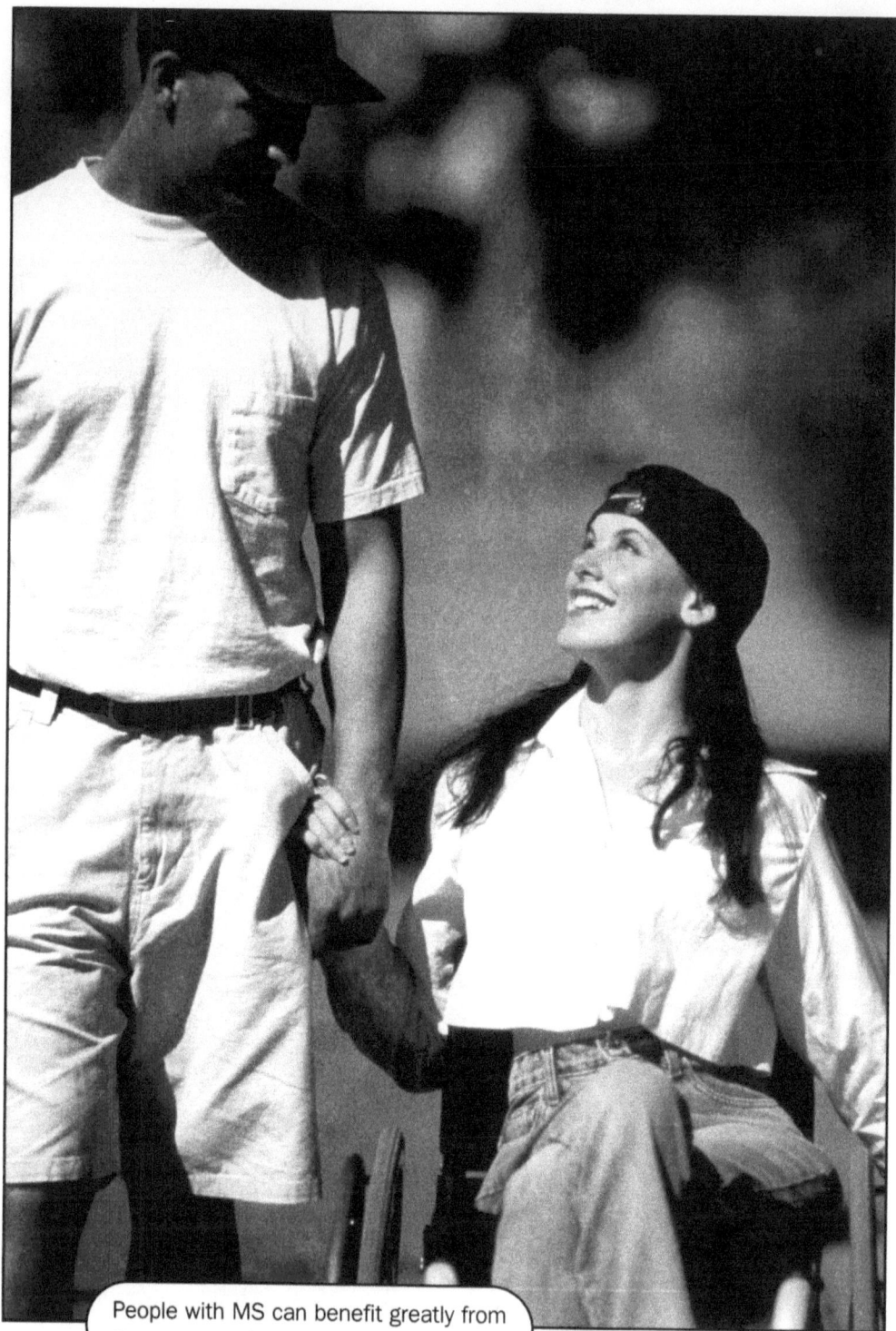

People with MS can benefit greatly from the support of family and friends.

Everything You Need to Know About

Multiple Sclerosis

Margaret J. Goldstein

The Rosen Publishing Group, Inc.
New York

The author would like to thank Carol Waldvogel for sharing her experiences, expertise, and invaluable insights into the lives of people with multiple sclerosis.

Published in 2001 by The Rosen Publishing Group, Inc.
29 East 21st Street, New York, NY 10010

Library of Congress Cataloging-in-Publication Data

Goldstein, Margaret J.
  Everything you need to know about multiple sclerosis / by Margaret J. Goldstein.
    p. cm.— (The need to know library)
Includes bibliographical references and index.
  ISBN: 978-1-4358-8671-1
  1. Multiple sclerosis—Juvenile literature. [1. Multiple sclerosis. 2. Diseases.] I. Title. II. Series.
  RC377 .G588 2000
  616.8'34—dc21

00-009604

Manufactured in the United States of America

Contents

Introduction

There it was in the mailbox: a big, fat envelope from the University of Colorado. Brett's heart raced. He had been accepted. He thought about attending school in Boulder—skiing, mountain biking, hiking in the Rockies. The university had a great premed program. But there was one problem—Boulder was 500 miles from his parents' house. Who was going to take care of his mom?

Brett's mom had multiple sclerosis. For as long as he could remember, he had been helping her fight the disease. Every spring, Brett's whole family took part in the MS Walk to raise money for medical research. Every summer, Brett rode in the MS Bike Tour, and ever since he had received his driver's license, he had been driving his mom to her doctors appointments.

Brett knew there was a good liberal arts school in his own city. Maybe he should just go to college near home. After all, what if his mom needed him? What if her MS got worse? Brett felt guilty and confused. What was more important: experiencing a new life or being there for his mother?

◆　◆　◆

Stephanie didn't have time for all these medical tests and procedures. She had applications to prepare, essays to write. If she was going to get into a top-level MBA program, she needed to focus. The competition for business school was fierce. She didn't want to deal with this MRI nonsense, and she was starting to wonder if the doctor at the university health clinic wasn't making something out of nothing.

Yes, she'd had a little numbness in her arms and legs. She'd tripped that one time. But it was probably just an accident—she'd never been very coordinated. Possible multiple sclerosis? That idea seemed ridiculous. She was only twenty-two years old. She'd never had anything worse than the flu in her life.

Stephanie wanted to get on with her future plans—business school, career, marriage, children.

"I don't think this doctor knows what he's talking about," she said to herself. But, deep down, she knew that something wasn't quite right.

◆　◆　◆

Kim found herself dreading the school play. It wasn't that she was afraid to perform. She loved the spotlight; the bigger the crowd, the better.

Actually, it was her father she was dreading— her father sitting in the audience. No way would he miss this play. He'd be there, front and center, watching the show from his electric scooter. At the reception afterward, he would want to talk to her friends and teachers, slurring his speech.

It was hard enough worrying about the regular pressures of high school, like boys, tests, grades, and SAT scores. Why did Kim have to worry about having a disabled parent, too? She knew it wasn't her father's fault. He had multiple sclerosis, and Kim helped him as much as she could. She loved him. But sometimes, even though she hated to admit it, she wished he would just stay at home.

Unanswered Questions

Teenagers need not be overly concerned with developing multiple sclerosis. It is a disease that usually does not strike until some time between your late twenties and early forties. Rarely, some young people like Stephanie develop MS as early as age twenty. Unfortunately, some young people, like Brett and Kim, do have to think about multiple sclerosis because they have parents who suffer from the disease.

People who develop multiple sclerosis, and their friends and family members, often have many questions and many fears. If you know someone with MS, you might not be sure how to help that person. You might even be afraid of getting the disease yourself. By educating yourself about MS, you'll be able to be less fearful and more helpful. Many people are involved in the effort to understand and treat MS, and to help those living with the disease. You can be one of them.

Chapter One | Medical Nuts and Bolts

Montel Williams leads an active and busy life. Viewers who watch *The Montel Williams Show* every day would probably never guess that the energetic, upbeat, and talkative host is sick. But, in August 1999, Williams revealed that he suffers from multiple sclerosis.

Williams was forty-two years old when doctors discovered that he had MS, but his symptoms began many years earlier. Occasionally, he had blurry vision. On and off, he felt pain in his feet and stiffness in his joints. At first, Williams shrugged off the trouble. He was young and athletic, after all. He jogged. He lifted weights. He wasn't going to let a few aches and pains slow him down. But, gradually, the pain grew worse. He began to feel weak. Finally, a doctor in California gave Williams a firm diagnosis: He had multiple sclerosis.

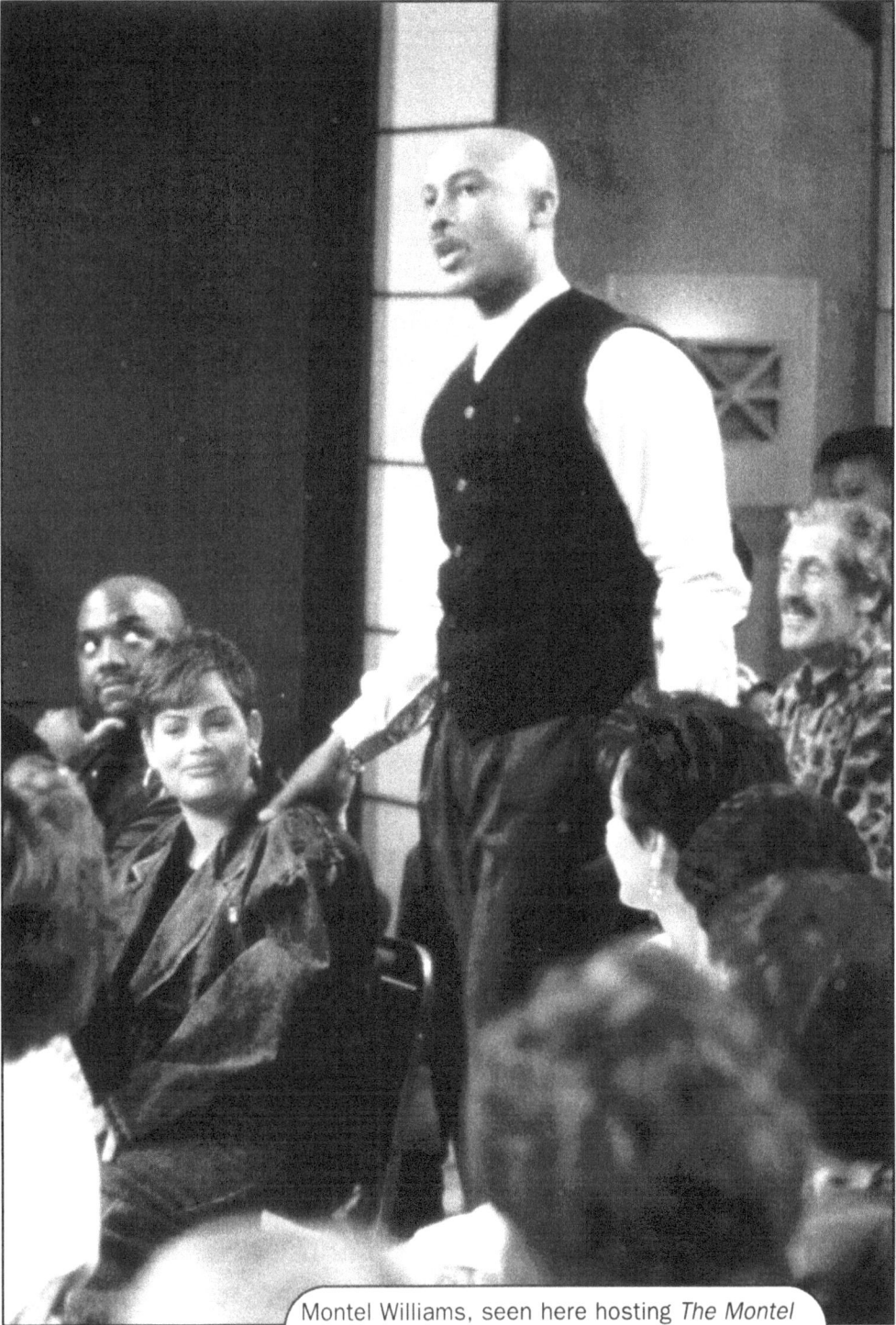

Montel Williams, seen here hosting *The Montel Williams Show*, has multiple sclerosis.

When you learn that you have a serious disease, it's normal to become upset, worried, and depressed. Williams did become depressed when he learned that he had multiple sclerosis, but he soon realized that something positive could come from his negative situation. By telling the public that he had MS, Williams would raise awareness and help others living with the disease. "I want to inspire people and show them that they can live and prosper with MS," he explained. "I want others affected by this disease to know that you can get out of bed."

Montel Williams is one of more than 300,000 Americans who suffers from multiple sclerosis. Other famous people with MS include comedian Richard Pryor and actors Annette Funicello (the original *Mickey Mouse Club*) and David Lander *(Laverne and Shirley)*. Multiple sclerosis affects different people in different ways. Symptoms might be mild or severe. They might grow worse or improve over time. Regardless of how the disease progresses, though, multiple sclerosis always begins in the same way—with the destruction of the myelin sheath, a protective covering around the nerves of the brain and spinal cord.

Communication Breakdown

The brain and the spinal cord make up the central nervous system, a kind of telecommunication network for the human body. Using a vast system of nerve cells, the brain sends and receives messages to and from the arms and legs, ears and eyes, heart and lungs, and every other part of the body. For instance, our eyes take in images of the things around us and send these images, via nerve cells, to the brain. In turn, the brain sends messages to the body, telling the legs to move, the mouth to speak, and the heart how often to beat. The spinal cord is the major pathway for carrying these messages to and from the brain.

A fatty substance called myelin surrounds and protects the nerves of the brain and spinal cord. Myelin functions similarly to insulation on electrical wires: It insures that messages between the brain and the body travel quickly and accurately. If parts of the myelin sheath (covering) are destroyed, messages can be interrupted or distorted. The brain might tell the legs to move, but that message won't get through correctly. Instead of walking smoothly, a person with MS might move slowly and awkwardly, and perhaps stumble.

Destruction of the myelin sheath, called demyelination, can occur anywhere in the central nervous system. Afterward, a scar or lesion—a hardened patch of tissue—might form over a damaged area. Another name for this scarring is *sclerosis*. A person with multiple areas of scarring on the myelin sheath is said to have multiple sclerosis.

A Variety of Symptoms

Scars on the myelin sheath can permanently interfere with motor functions, such as walking, and sensory functions, such as vision. The symptoms of MS vary from person to person, depending on where the scars occur. Common symptoms include the following:

+ Weakness

+ Numbness

+ Tremors

+ Fatigue

+ Pain

+ Poor coordination

+ Loss of balance

+ Difficulty walking

+ Difficulty speaking

+ Loss of bladder or bowel control

+ Visual problems

+ Paralysis

In addition, some people with MS suffer from cognitive, or thinking, problems. Symptoms can include memory loss, mood swings, and difficulties in problem solving. This is because MS attacks the brain and therefore affects the systems we use to remember things, feel emotions, and reason.

The primary, or main, symptoms of MS can also lead to secondary symptoms. These are complications that arise from the effects of the primary symptoms. For instance, difficulty in walking can lead to inactivity and then to decreased bone density. As a result, a person with multiple sclerosis might be more likely to break bones than a person who doesn't have the disease.

Tertiary (third-tier) symptoms are social and emotional complications that arise from primary and secondary symptoms. Examples are depression and the loss of job skills. For instance, imagine a chef who develops multiple sclerosis. Vision problems and tremors might interfere with his or her ability to read recipes, measure ingredients precisely, and use knives and other kitchen tools. Eventually, the chef might have to abandon his or her career altogether.

A Progressive Disease

As Montel Williams discovered, MS doesn't just show up in full force overnight. In fact, Williams experienced mild symptoms of multiple sclerosis for more than fifteen years before doctors finally diagnosed the disease. He learned that he has relapsing-remitting MS, which means that his symptoms come and go over time. He has relapses, also called exacerbations or flare-ups, followed by long periods of remission, or partial recovery. He is usually able to work normally, with little disruption of his talk-show duties. Relapsing-remitting MS is the most common form of the disease.

For many people with relapsing-remitting MS, symptoms grow steadily worse over time. Flare-ups begin to occur more often. Remission becomes less frequent. The person is then said to have secondary-progressive MS. A third form of the disease, primary-progressive MS (also called chronic-progressive) is progressive from the start—symptoms begin to worsen right away, and remission is limited. Primary-progressive MS is the least common form of the disease.

Multiple sclerosis is not a fatal disease. People with MS generally live 90 to 95 percent of the normal life span. However, as the disease progresses, it can cause great disability. Those who experience mild symptoms at first—the occasional tremor or numbness—might, over many years, lose their ability to speak, walk, and work normally. Because MS affects the brain as well as the body, people with MS might also experience memory loss, difficulty reasoning, mood swings, and other psychological problems. MS is also an unpredictable disease; its symptoms can worsen, lessen, or change over time. One of the most frustrating problems facing people with MS is uncertainty. They never know when flare-ups might occur and what form they might take.

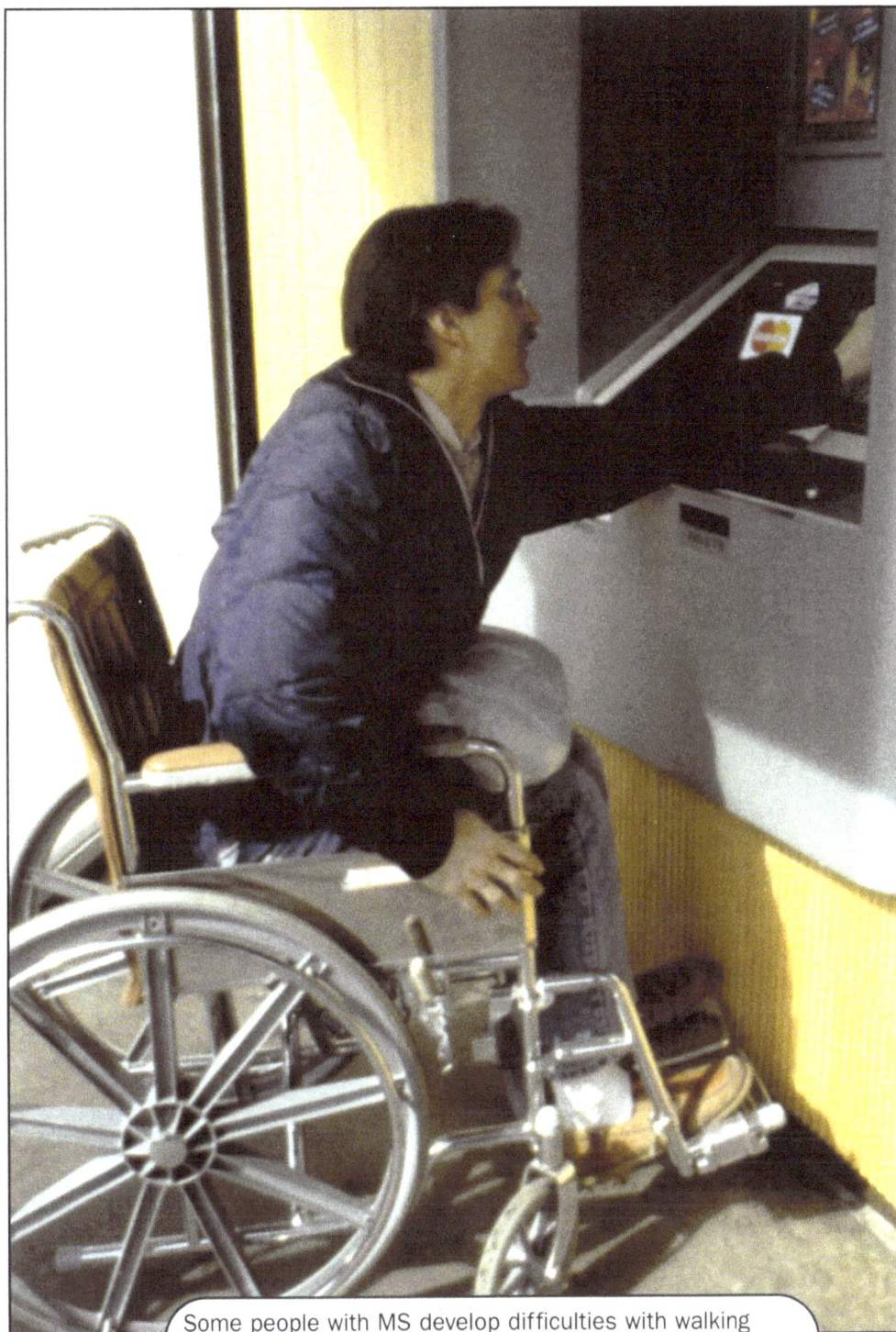

Some people with MS develop difficulties with walking and need to rely on wheelchairs, canes, and other devices.

People diagnosed with MS often fear that they'll lose the ability to walk and that they'll eventually be confined to a bed or a wheelchair. Many people with MS do have difficulty walking. Some of them use canes, walkers, and other devices for assistance. They might use electric scooters or wheelchairs for some activities. But most people with MS (two out of three) remain ambulatory over their lifetime, meaning that they are able to walk, although they often need assistance.

The keys to living well with MS are proper medical treatment, physical therapy and assistance, and the emotional support of friends and family.

Chapter Two | Who Gets MS and Why?

*P*aula and Heather had always been close. They attended the same college, shared secrets, even shared an apartment for a while. Then, when she was twenty-seven, Heather learned that she had multiple sclerosis. Paula couldn't help feeling a little weird around Heather after that. After all, Heather was just a year older than Paula, and she already had to walk with a cane. Paula knew that MS wasn't contagious, but she still began spending less and less time with her friend. When they were together, Paula was afraid to mention Heather's condition. She even felt a little guilty about her own good health. Paula wanted to help Heather, but she wasn't sure how.

Finally, Heather broke the ice. "Join me in the walkathon to raise money for research into MS *and the search for better treatments—maybe even a cure," Heather suggested. Paula agreed to go, but the sight of people in wheelchairs and electric scooters depressed her at first. Then Paula noticed something else: lots of kids and families walking together. Lots of cheering and laughing—everyone pulling together for a common cause. All of a sudden, Paula didn't feel so uncomfortable around Heather anymore. As they walked, the two friends talked about Heather's fears and the challenges of having MS. Paula asked lots of questions and did a lot of listening. She realized how she could help Heather the most: by being the same friend she had always been.*

Heather and Paula, setting off on the annual MS Walk, are just two links in an enormous chain of people with MS, their friends and families, doctors, medical researchers, educators, counselors, and therapists who are all working toward a common goal: to better understand what causes MS and to find effective treatments and, eventually, a cure.

The search for a cure and treatments for any disease begins with medical research. But, despite decades of study, multiple sclerosis is still something of a mystery to researchers. Many questions about the causes of MS remain unanswered. That's not to

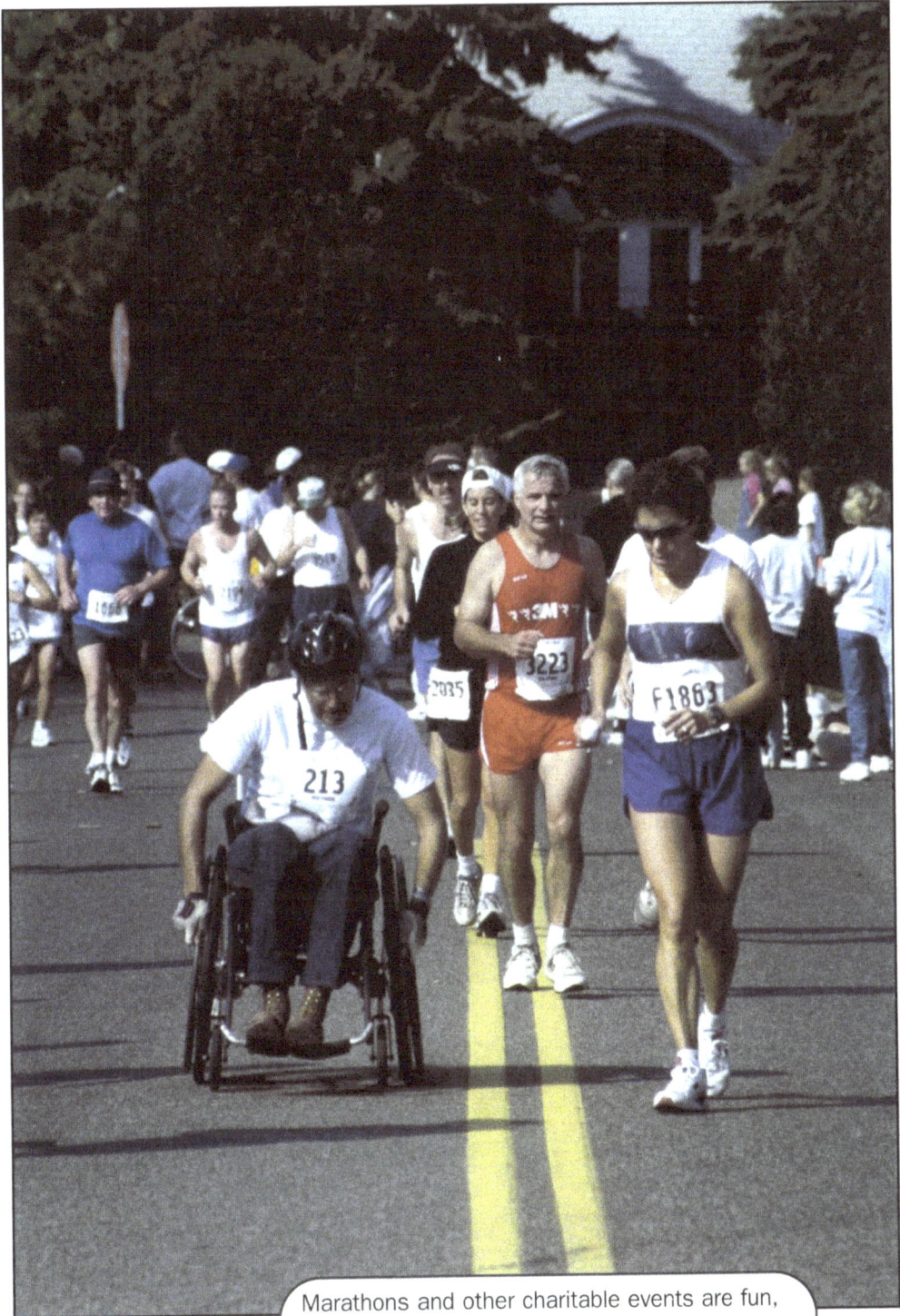

Marathons and other charitable events are fun, and they help to raise money for MS research.

say that doctors and researchers know nothing about the causes of MS. In fact, researchers are fairly sure that it's an autoimmune response that causes destruction of the myelin sheath. This means that the immune system, the bodily system that normally defends the body against infection, actually attacks and destroys myelin. In a way, MS is the result of the body attacking itself.

What doctors don't know, however, is *why* the immune system attacks the myelin sheath. What triggers the attack? What makes a person likely to get multiple sclerosis? Why do some people get multiple sclerosis and not others?

Trends and Statistics

To answer these questions, scientists must first study people who have MS to determine what, if anything, they have in common. Although anyone can get multiple sclerosis, some people are more prone to the disease than others. Here's what scientists have found:

- Those with a close relative with MS (a parent or sibling) are more likely to develop the disease than the average person.

- Whites (especially those of northern European descent) are more likely to develop MS than are blacks, Asians, Hispanics, and Native Americans.

- Women are twice as likely as men to get MS.

- People who live in cold, northern areas are more likely to develop the disease than people from other places.

Unraveling the Mystery

What do these facts tell us? A lot, actually. First of all, MS might be linked to genetics—biological traits that are shared by family members and passed from parents to children. Studies show that the average person has a 1 in 1,000 chance of developing multiple sclerosis. But if you have a parent or sibling with the disease, your chance of developing MS increases to between 1 in 100 and 1 in 50. If you have an identical twin with multiple sclerosis, then your chance is even greater: 1 in 3. The fact that multiple sclerosis occurs more often in whites of northern European descent than in other ethnic groups provides further evidence of a possible link between MS and genetics, since certain genes are more common among specific ethnic or racial groups.

But genes don't tell the whole story. More than 80 percent of the people who develop MS do not have a parent or sibling with the disease. And identical twins share all the same genes, yet one twin might develop MS while the other might not. Genetics, it appears, is only part of the MS mystery.

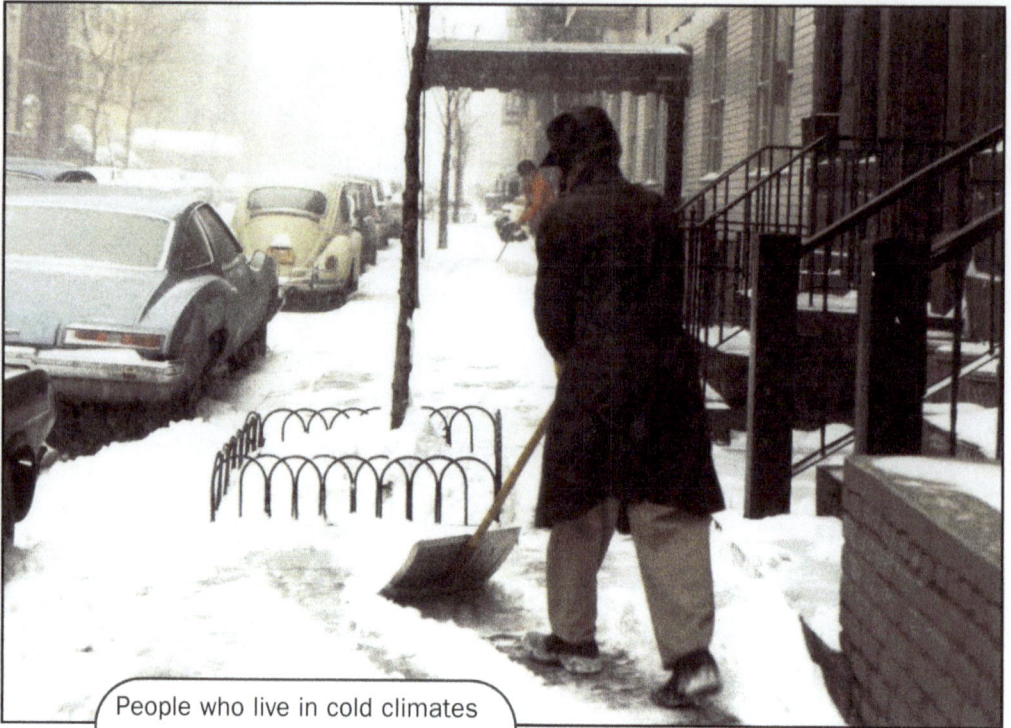

People who live in cold climates are more likely to develop MS.

Environment plays another part. People from cold, northern climates are more likely to develop MS than those from warm places. But if a child moves from a cold place to a warm place before age fifteen, his or her chance of developing MS goes down. What is it about cold climates that increases a person's chance of developing MS? Scientists don't know. Why do women get MS more often than men? Another mystery.

Finally, some researchers believe that a virus might trigger the autoimmune response that causes destruction of myelin in the central nervous system. Putting all of the theories and statistics together, scientists have made an educated guess about what causes MS. They believe that some people might be genetically prone to the disease and that exposure to a virus or an environmental influence can trigger an autoimmune response in these people, destroying myelin and leading to multiple sclerosis.

Sound complicated? It is—and doctors have a long way to go before they fully understand MS and its causes. Ideally, of course, all the research and testing will lead to a cure for MS. But short of finding a cure, doctors hope that their efforts will lead to more effective treatments for MS and drugs that will slow the progress of the disease.

Chapter Three | Diagnosis and Treatment

David was stunned. The doctor's words all ran together into one confusing jumble: "Relapsing" what? "Myelin" something or other? "Magnetic resonance" . . . what was that again? There was only one term that David understood quite clearly: "Multiple sclerosis." The words rang in his head like a bell.

The doctor had been carefully monitoring David's symptoms for months now. She had done her work, run through all the tests, and double-checked her results. But David's work was just beginning.

Multiple sclerosis can take a great toll on physical health. A short walk around the block might seem like a marathon to a person with MS. Simple tasks such as dressing and combing your hair—even swallowing food—might eventually become difficult.

A variety of treatments—drugs and therapies—can alleviate the symptoms of MS and improve day-to-day life for people living with the disease. Good medical and physical care is key. But before people can get that care, they have to know they have MS in the first place.

A Difficult Diagnosis

MS might begin with a little numbness. A mysterious pain that shows up and disappears. But who hasn't experienced the occasional ache or pain? Most of us don't run to the doctor every time we feel a slight ache, which explains why multiple sclerosis often goes undetected, especially early on. Many people shrug off the early signs of MS and go forward with life as normal.

Over time, though, symptoms might become more frequent and harder to ignore. But even after people seek medical treatment, an MS diagnosis could be a long way off because multiple sclerosis is difficult to pin down. Doctors can't always tell whether symptoms such as pain, fatigue, tremors, or loss of balance are due to MS or to a different disease or disorder. At first, a doctor might not even think to check for MS. He or she might assume that mild symptoms will pass or even tell the patient, "It's all in your head."

For an official MS diagnosis, a person must have experienced at least two flare-ups at least one month apart and must show evidence of more than one area of scarring on the myelin sheath. To examine the myelin sheath, doctors usually use a technique called MRI (magnetic resonance imaging). MRI uses radio waves and a magnet to create a special picture of the brain. But even if MRI reveals scarring on the myelin sheath, doctors know that the damage might stem from another disease besides MS. Also, if scarring occurs on the patient's spinal cord instead of the brain, MRI results might look normal—even though the patient in fact has MS.

Because of these complicating factors, doctors do not rely on MRI alone to diagnose MS. They interview patients about symptoms. They also conduct neurological exams, testing the patient's memory, balance, coordination, vision, and reflexes. They might also use tests called evoked potentials, which detect a slowing down of messages in the brain. They sometimes analyze spinal fluid, looking for evidence of abnormal immune responses.

Even when many test results point to MS, doctors can't always be certain in their diagnoses. Until they rule out other likely diseases, doctors might say that a person has "possible MS" or "probable MS." For patients, not knowing for sure whether or not they have MS can be unsettling and frustrating. Some people are

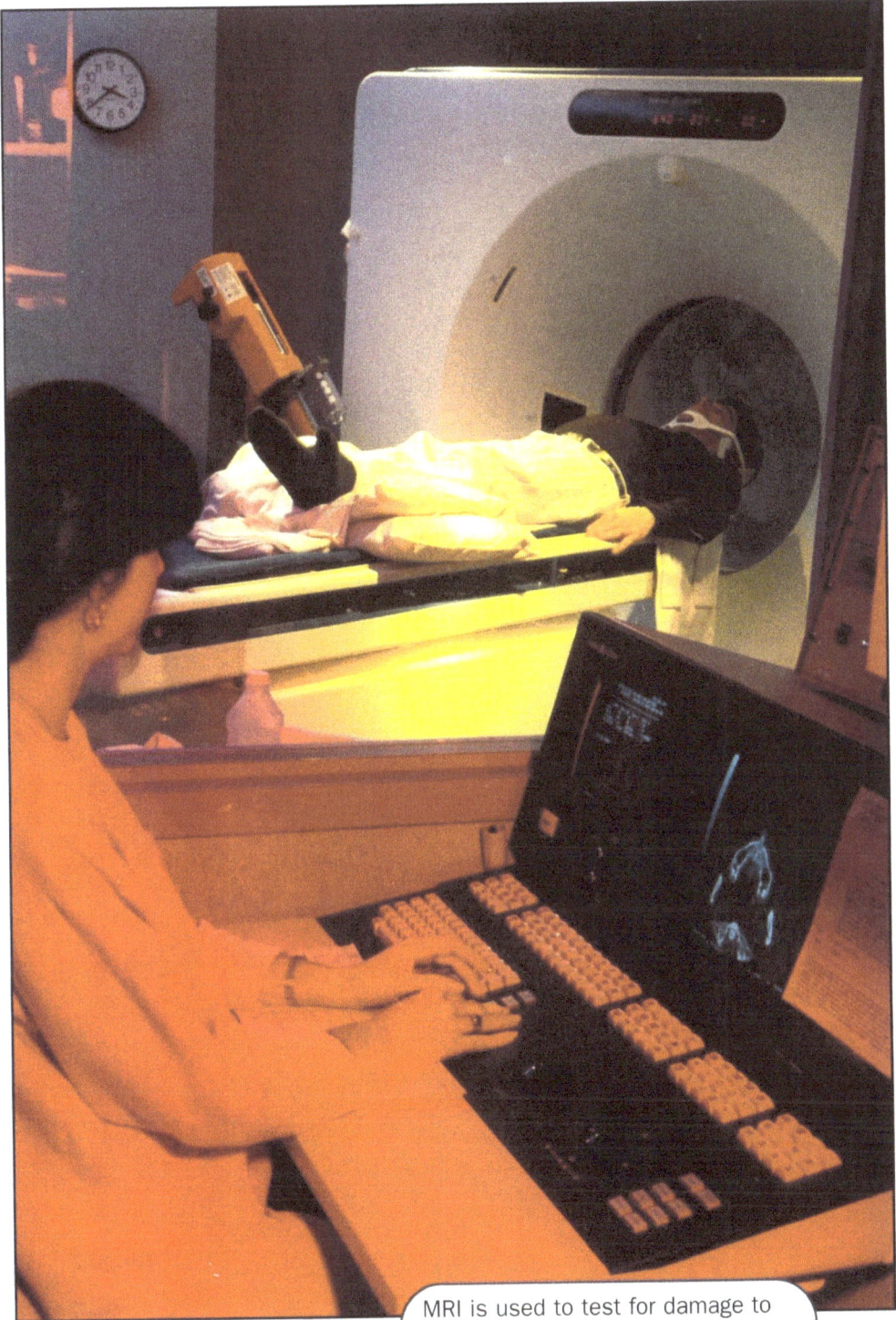

MRI is used to test for damage to the brain's myelin sheath.

actually relieved when they finally learn they have MS. Then they can stop wondering what's wrong and begin treating the illness.

Physical Care

While there is no cure for MS, three drugs approved by the FDA (Food and Drug Administration) have been shown to slow the course of the disease. These drugs, Avonex, Betaseron, and Copaxone, can lessen the frequency and severity of flare-ups and slow destruction of the myelin sheath. Other medications relieve specific symptoms, such as pain, fatigue, and bladder problems.

Many people with MS benefit from exercise. "I would urge you to exercise each day," advises one longtime MS patient, speaking to those newly diagnosed with the disease. "Do not overexert but go a little further every day. You will be amazed at what this will do for your spirits, your energy level, and your strength."

Health care specialists recommend stretching to counteract muscle stiffness and aerobics for overall fitness. Lifting small weights builds strength and improves muscle tone. Swimming is a good way for people with MS to exercise, since water helps support the body during exercise sessions.

Some people with MS exercise with the help of physical therapists, who can recommend specific stretches and exercises to improve strength, coordination, balance,

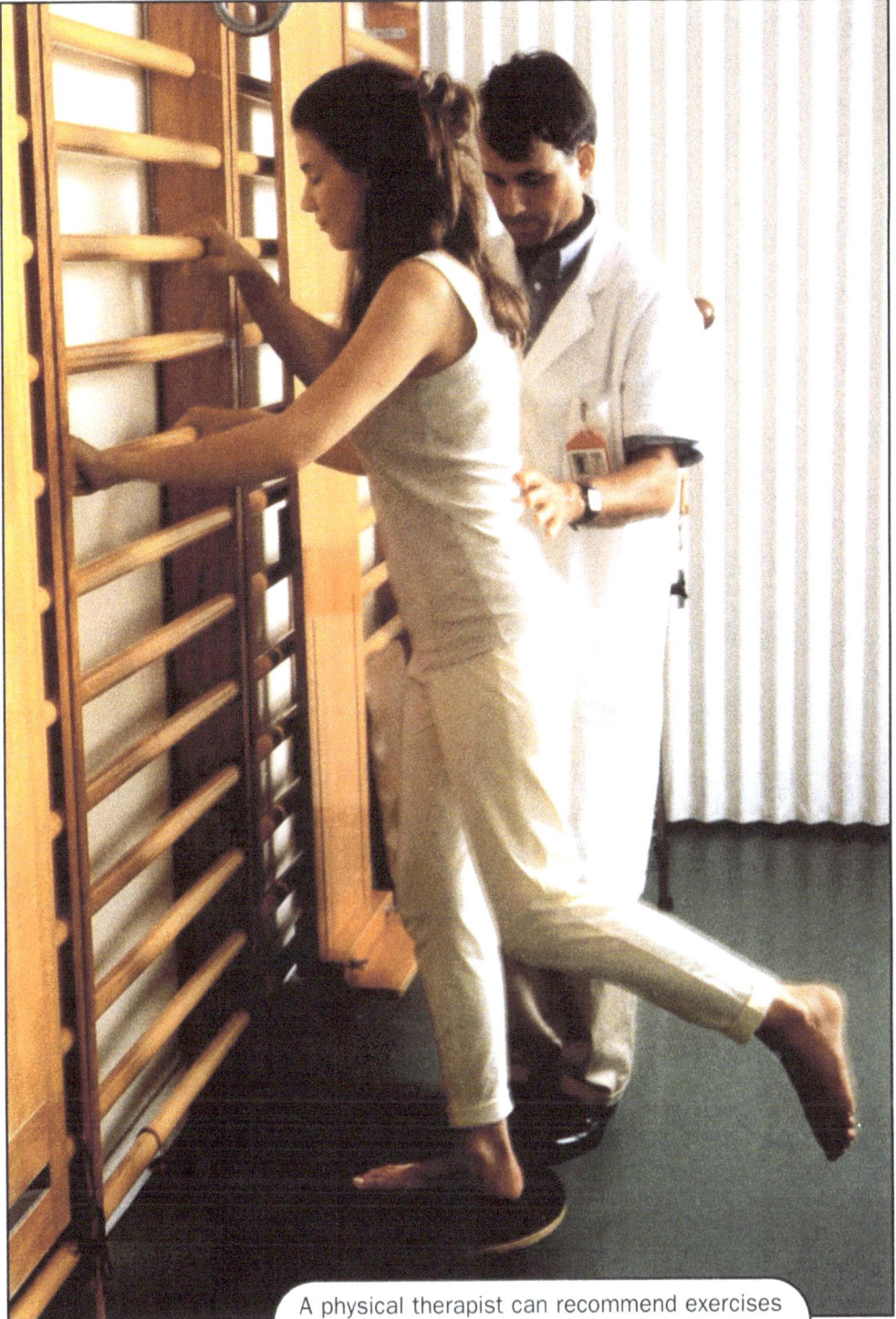

A physical therapist can recommend exercises that improve coordination and strength.

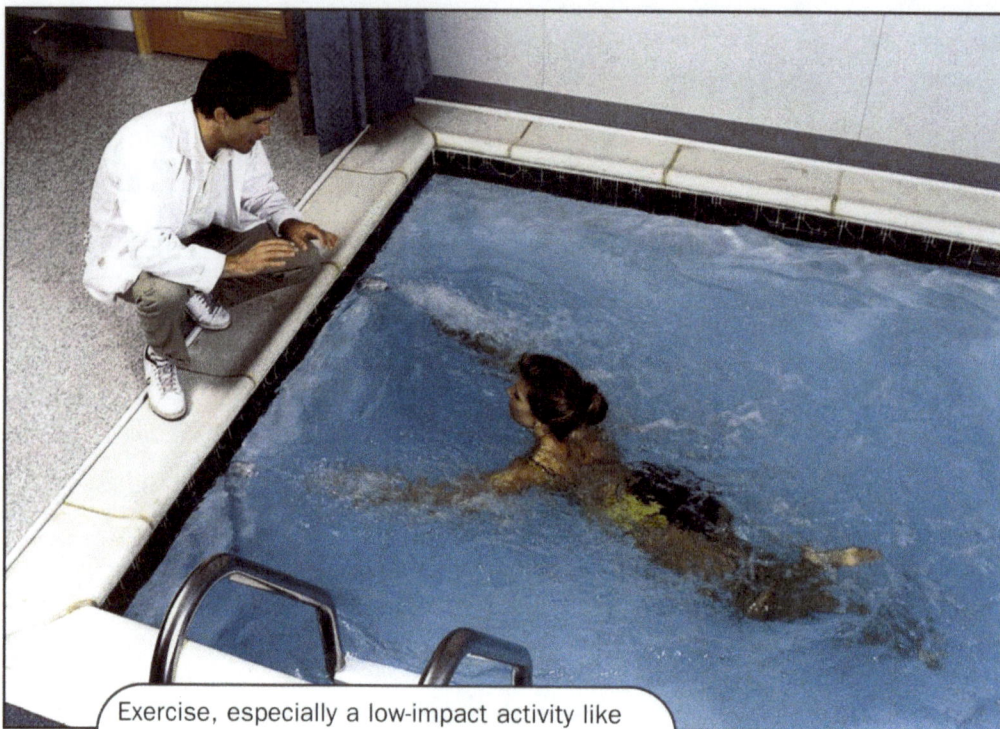
Exercise, especially a low-impact activity like swimming, is beneficial for people with MS.

and flexibility. Occupational therapists help patients learn new ways to perform day-to-day tasks, such as dressing or cooking, while seated in a wheelchair.

Heat can temporarily intensify fatigue and other symptoms of MS, so patients must be sure to stay cool. Cool baths, cold drinks, and ice packs can help relieve symptoms. Air-conditioning at home and in the car is a must on hot days.

In some ways, the programs doctors recommend to help people with MS stay healthy—exercise, stretching, and relaxation—are no different from the typical health advice doctors give to everyone. Similarly, people with MS are advised to eat a well-balanced and nutritious diet, watch their weight, and avoid cigarettes and alcohol.

Chapter Four

Treating the Spirit

*L*isa did the dishes a lot. Lisa did the laundry a lot. Lisa cooked a lot. Once, Lisa even made Thanksgiving dinner for eight people when her mother had a bad flare-up the day before. In fact, Lisa figured she could cook just about any kind of food, solve just about any dilemma. There was only one problem she couldn't fix—her mother's multiple sclerosis.

There was no way around the facts. Lisa's mother was sometimes too weak to leave her chair. She sometimes forgot her doctors appointments, and Lisa had to reschedule them. It was almost as if Lisa was the parent to her own mother. She was only fifteen, but she felt like she'd barely had a childhood at all.

MS changes lives—not only the lives of those who are diagnosed with the disease but also the lives of their families. As MS progresses, household chores and activities such as driving can become difficult to perform. Partners, children, and other family members might have to pick up the slack. Even very young children might have to change their routines and responsibilities to help a parent who has MS.

Reactions to an MS Diagnosis

MS is typically diagnosed between the ages of twenty and forty. For a previously healthy person in this age range, the diagnosis can come as a real shock. "I was just twenty-nine when the doctor told me it was MS," says Brooke. "I was like, you've got to be kidding. I was numb." Some people refuse to believe the MS diagnosis altogether. They might visit doctor after doctor, looking for a different explanation for their symptoms. They might try to ignore the symptoms, refusing to use a cane, for instance, even when walking is difficult.

Fear is another common reaction to the MS diagnosis. Will I become disabled? Will I lose my independence? Will I be in pain? All these fears commonly run through the mind of a person newly diagnosed with MS.

Anger is yet another possible response. Some people feel angry with their doctors. They "blame the messenger," so to speak, for giving them the bad news. Others direct their anger at no one in particular, just at the unfair situation.

Finally, it is typical for people diagnosed with MS—or any serious illness—to experience sadness and depression. In truth, an MS diagnosis means that life will likely become more difficult. A person with MS might eventually have to give up favorite hobbies, sports, even a career. The sense of loss can be powerful.

"Your first job is to take control of your emotional well-being," advises one woman with MS. She cautions those newly diagnosed with the disease, "Don't let negative emotions take you for a ride."

Ongoing Struggles

Often, people who suffer only mild symptoms of MS handle the diagnosis with ease. Especially in the early stages, people with MS might feel well most of the time. They don't look sick, and few people other than family and friends even know they have MS. These people often proceed with jobs and social activities with little disruption. But if symptoms worsen over time, and ordinary tasks begin to get more difficult, these same people might experience the feelings of anger, sadness, and depression they at first avoided.

The progression of MS varies from person to person. Some people experience only mild symptoms throughout their lifetime, while others become severely disabled.

Flare-ups (exacerbations) can occur without warning. Similarly, the situation might improve all of a sudden— with fewer flare-ups and longer periods of remission. For people with MS and their families, this unpredictability can be extremely frustrating.

Just as MS symptoms vary from person to person, emotional struggles vary as well. A person with MS who lives alone might feel increasingly isolated, since MS can decrease mobility and make it hard to leave the house and socialize. Parents with MS might feel guilty about not being able to give their all to their children. They might feel helpless, or even worthless, if they are unable to work, cook dinner, or drive their kids to after-school activities. People who once lived active, athletic lives might become irritable or short-tempered as MS decreases their physical abilities. Those who were once very outgoing might withdraw from group activities, because they don't want friends to see their new physical limits or to feel sorry for them. Stress is common for people with MS and their families, as everyone has to compromise and change their routines to take on new roles and responsibilities.

The mental health effects of MS only add to other emotional problems. Mood swings can be a direct result of lesions (scarring) on the brain. Memory loss is another primary symptom related to destruction of the myelin sheath.

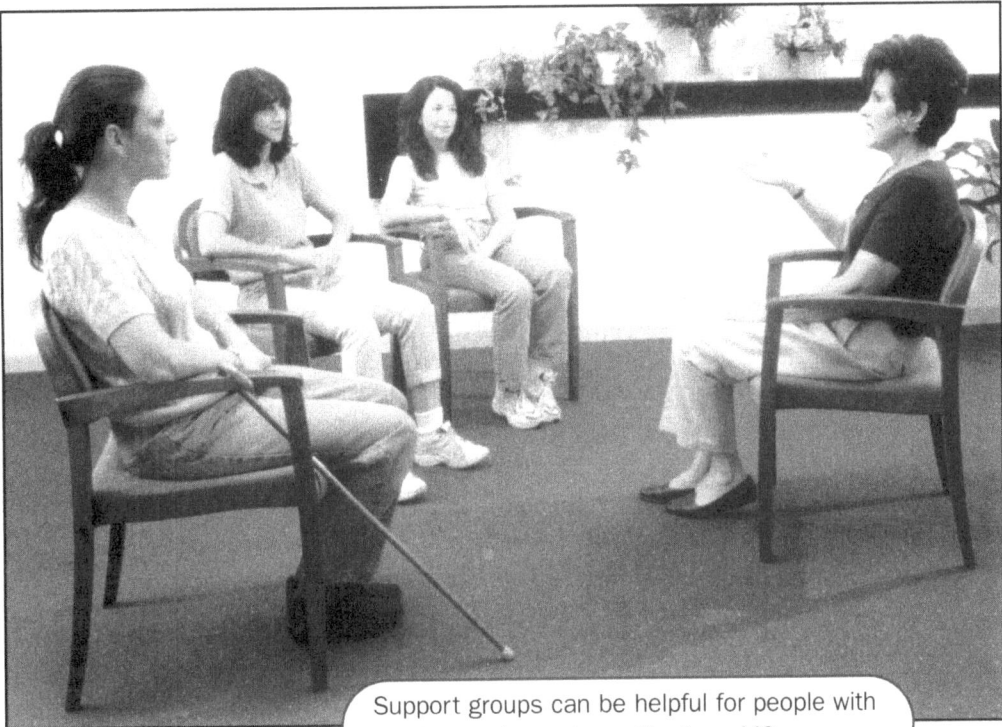
Support groups can be helpful for people with family members who suffer from MS.

In the face of very real and difficult emotional struggles, health care providers recommend that people with MS seek out individual and family counseling, support groups made up of other MS patients, and honest communication with family and friends. In some cases, doctors prescribe antidepressant medications to help patients through times of extra difficulty.

Kids and Their Parents

"When I was nine, Mom came to my soccer game in her wheelchair," Kevin remembers. *"Some kid said, 'Who's the kooky lady in the wheelchair?' and I pretended I didn't know. Later, I asked my mom not to come to games*

anymore. I feel bad about that now because I know it hurt her."

Kevin, like many kids who have a parent with MS, must balance a range of emotions. Kids are typically worried about fitting in. They don't want to be seen as weird or different. And they certainly don't want to have "weird" parents. Kevin felt embarrassed by his mother's disability, but at the same time, he loved her and worried about her. He felt guilty for asking her to stay away from games. For kids with parents with MS, this kind of emotional conflict arises all the time.

Even very young children are affected by their parents' MS. Kids as young as three or four might have to help with the dishes, get dressed on their own, or pick up their own toys if a mother or father isn't able to move easily. Young children, especially, can't understand a complicated disease like MS. "Is my mother going to die?" a child might wonder. "If I'm extra good and clean my room, will my father get better?" another child might ask. Counselors advise parents to talk openly with children about their fears about MS. If negative feelings go unaddressed, children might express them by misbehaving in school, withdrawing from other kids, or acting aggressively.

Older kids, including teenagers, face other problems. "When you're in junior high, you have your reputation, your image. You want to be cool," explains one teen.

Kids might avoid inviting friends over for dinner or might discourage parents with MS from visiting school. They might even feel angry or resentful toward a parent with MS—because a kid who's needed at home for cooking, cleaning, or running errands will probably have less time for sports and social activities.

Kids who take on extra responsibilities—such as helping care for a parent with MS—sometimes seem to grow up faster than other children. They might make an extra effort to be well behaved and to get good grades in school so they don't put further burdens on their families. They might put their parents' needs before their own. For instance, some teenagers hesitate to apply to college far from home, worried that a parent with MS might need them nearby.

Beneath this "grown-up" exterior, though, a child whose parent has MS might feel frightened, sad, or angry. Counselors advise kids to talk openly about these emotions, not only with their parents but also with their siblings and friends. Many teens find help in peer support groups made up of other kids who have parents with MS.

Partners and Spouses

Partners of people with MS also face emotional struggles. Some spouses feel more like health care workers than equal partners, especially if the person with MS suffers physical decline. "I don't have MS, but I've been quite depressed," explains one woman whose husband has MS. "All we talk about are doctors and medicines. There is no fun anymore, just arguments and misunderstandings."

Indeed, some of the emotional distress that affects people with MS is likely to affect their partners, too. Depression, anger, stress, and fear are common. As the physically healthy person, the partner must usually take on more responsibilities for child care, household chores, and supporting the family. Many spouses feel resentful of the extra demands on their time and energy. They might also feel bad about enjoying favorite hobbies, sports, and activities while the partner with MS can no longer join in.

Many people with MS note that their sexual and romantic lives suffer because of the disease. There are many reasons for this. First, MS attacks the nervous system, the place where sexual feelings begin. Many people with MS report a loss of sensation in their sexual organs. Bladder problems such as incontinence can add discomfort or embarrassment to sexual situations. Fatigue and pain might add more barriers to romance.

Emotional problems compound the physical ones. For instance, stress and depression can reduce a person's sex drive. And people with MS may lose self-confidence. They may feel that their physical disabilities make them less attractive to sexual partners. Doctors recommend

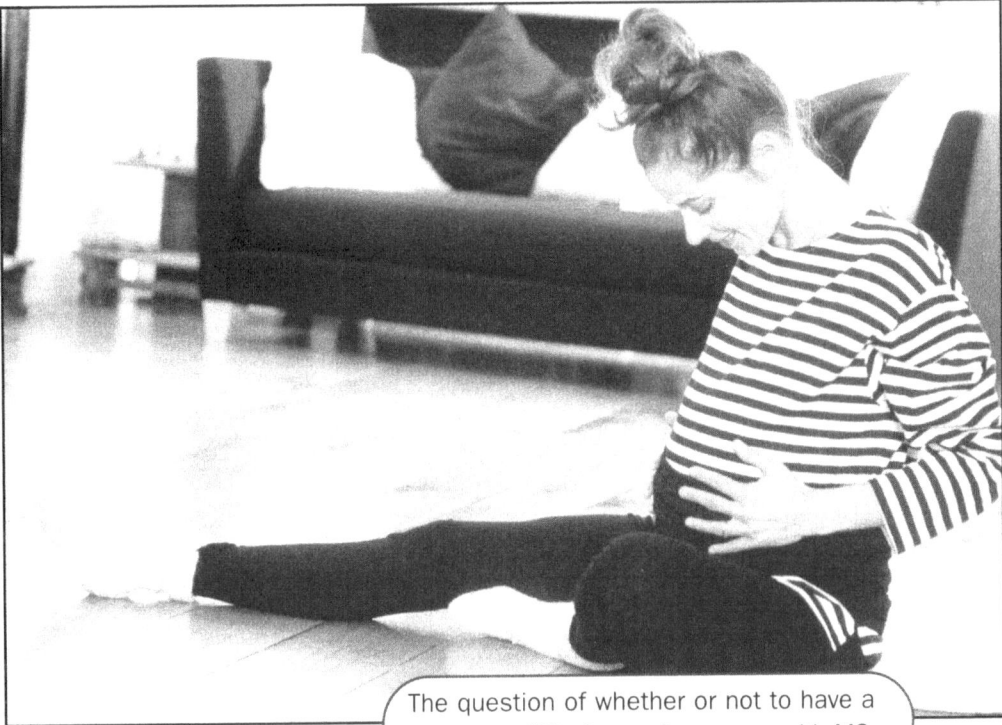

The question of whether or not to have a child is a difficult one for women with MS.

honest communication between partners regarding sexual problems, as well as counseling, medicines to relieve symptoms, and sexual aids.

MS strikes people "in their prime"—between the ages of twenty and forty. Many people newly diagnosed with MS have recently been married. Some have recently had children or plan to start a family. Should a woman with MS have a child? While doctors believe that pregnancy and childbirth do not affect the overall course of MS, they note that exacerbations might increase after delivery. In addition, MS can complicate pregnancy. For instance, pregnancy often causes fatigue and difficulties walking, even for those in good health, so these problems are naturally increased in women with MS.

Doctors advise people with MS—both male and female—to think carefully about how they will support and care for a child should one parent become severely disabled. They warn women with MS about the physical demands of looking after a baby. For many people, though, the joys of raising children greatly outweigh such concerns.

Chapter Five | MS in the Home and Workplace

As usual, Bob pulled into a handicapped parking spot in front of the grocery store. He walked slowly to the line of shopping carts and wheeled one toward the door—the cart was as good as a cane for giving him support when he walked through the store.

Then he heard a hostile voice: "You've got a lot of nerve using that parking space—that's for disabled people," a woman shouted at him. Bob turned and pointed to the handicap permit hanging prominently in the windshield of his car. "Oh," the woman said, acting embarrassed. "Sorry. But you don't look sick ... What's wrong with you anyway?"

Think about the little tasks you do all day long: carrying a bag of groceries, typing at the computer, flipping on light switches, making a quick drive to the supermarket, walking from class to class at school, jumping up to answer the phone, buttoning your shirt. These tasks probably don't cause you much trouble. You probably don't think about all the bones, nerves, and muscles that have to work together to make each movement smooth and precise or how your eyes guide you as you go.

If you had MS, though, these ordinary tasks might seem extraordinary. A small inconvenience—a bicycle blocking the sidewalk, for instance—might look like a giant roadblock to you. You might even have to give up driving because of vision problems—no more quick trips to the grocery store. What can people with MS do to cope when ordinary life becomes difficult? In short, they must adapt.

Walking the Walk

"Putting one foot in front of the other is a remarkable, technical feat we ordinarily take for granted," says Dr. George Kraft, professor of rehabilitation medicine at the University of Washington. But many people with MS don't take walking for granted. For them, a walk from the living room to the kitchen can be an exhausting trip.

Exercise and stretching can help, but many people with MS find that mobility devices such as walkers, canes, and braces give them the additional support they need—an extra "leg to stand on," so to speak. Many people with MS are reluctant to use a wheelchair or an electric scooter. They don't want to be seen as disabled. In fact, many MS patients who use wheelchairs and scooters can actually walk. They use the wheeled devices for covering long distances—a trip through the zoo, for instance—and to save strength for other tasks. "A wheelchair is actually liberating because it enables you to do more," says Dr. Kraft. People who use wheelchairs and scooters walk more easily, he explains, because they don't tire themselves out trying to walk everywhere.

Design Specialists

People with MS often become masters at redesigning their homes to accommodate their special physical needs. They might widen doorways to make room for wheelchairs or walkers. They might lower countertops for easy reach from a scooter. They might install all sorts of gadgets and devices to help make life at home easier. These devices can include:

- Sliding doors
- Lever-style door handles
- Grab bars in bathrooms and bedrooms
- Hospital-style hi-low beds

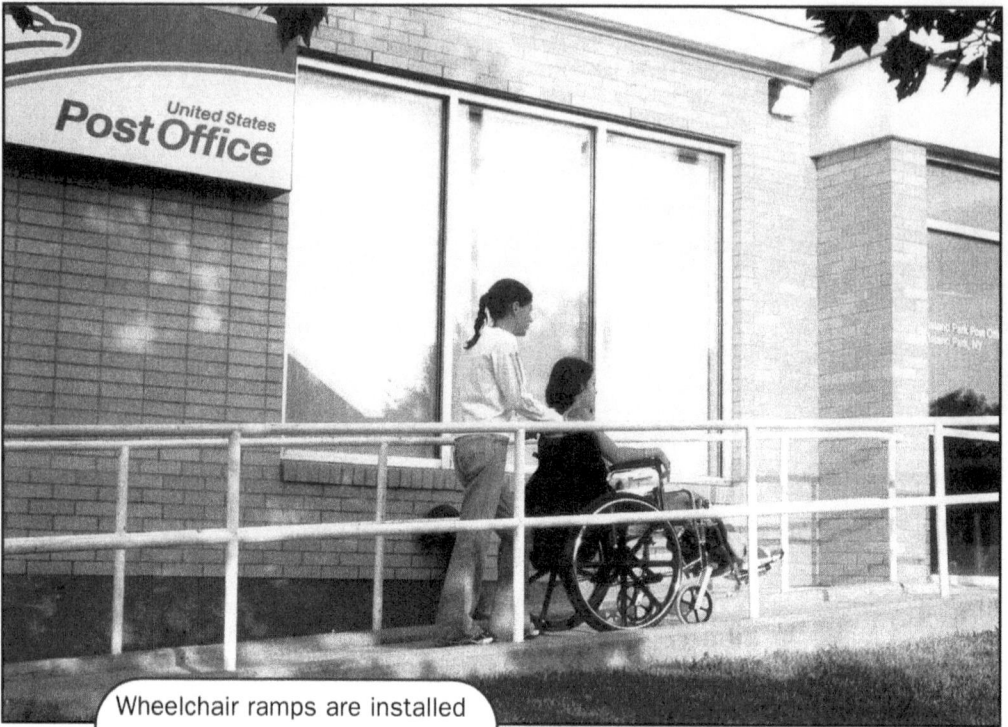

Wheelchair ramps are installed outside many public buildings.

- Wheelchair ramps

- Stair-climbing chairs

- Handbrakes for cars

- Grooming and dressing aids

- Magnifying devices (for poor vision)

- Computers that respond to voice commands

- Remote controls for lights, fans, and other appliances

You've probably seen wheelchair ramps, handicapped parking spots, wide checkout aisles, and large toilet stalls with grab bars at schools, stores, restaurants, and other public buildings. Though not always available, these accommodations can make a big difference to people with MS (and other disabilities). Without them, going shopping, running errands, and attending social events can become nearly impossible, especially for a person who uses a wheelchair or an electric scooter.

Many people with MS become very organized. They plan ahead. They make sure that the phone is always nearby and preprogrammed with emergency numbers. They get rid of unnecessary clutter and store important items within easy reach. People with cognitive problems find that appointment books, to-do lists, electronic organizers, and calendars can help make up for slips in memory or a decline in problem-solving skills. Often, physical and occupational therapists help people with MS find the best devices and systems for adapting to their new limitations.

Help at Home

Sometimes gadgets and systems are not enough. Sometimes people with MS, especially those who live alone, might need help with such household tasks as cooking, driving, bill paying, shopping, laundry—even dressing and bathing. Some people will need a visiting nurse to administer medicines or change catheter bags (for those with bladder problems) or a visiting physical or occupational therapist to assist them in exercising.

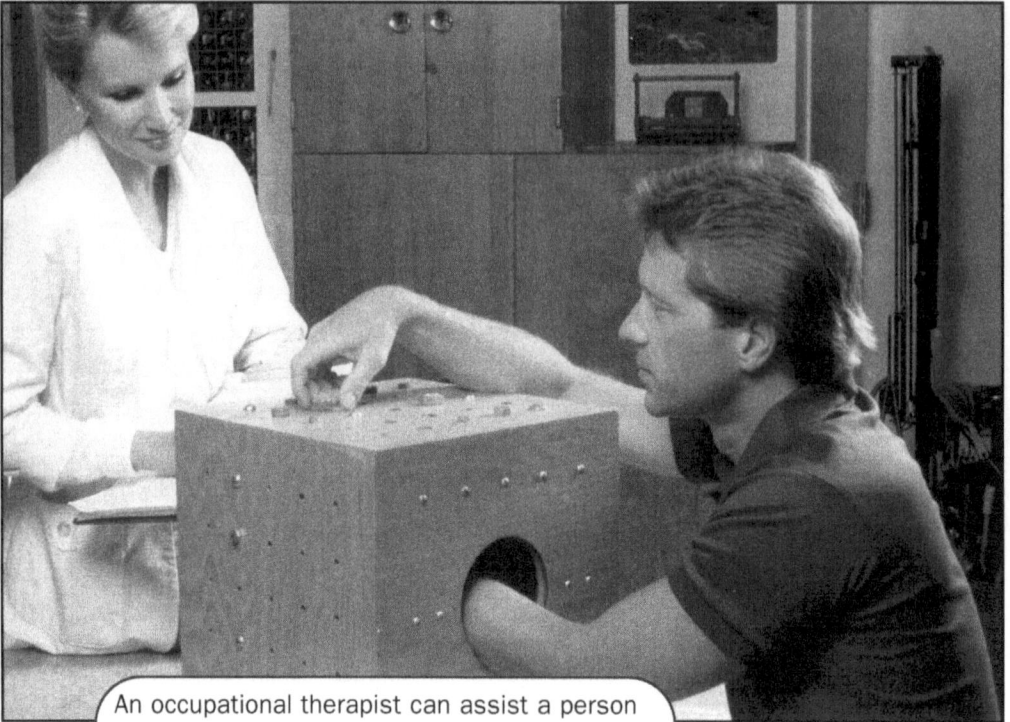

An occupational therapist can assist a person with MS in developing his or her coordination.

Many people with MS resist the fact that they need help. Naturally, most people, sick or not, don't want to lose independence, privacy, and a sense of control over their own lives. Nevertheless, home help is sometimes a necessity. Professional assistance can also take a great burden off family members, who are not usually trained to handle the medical problems that might arise as MS progresses. In the event of severe disability, people with MS might need to move to a nursing home, but this is generally not the case.

On the Job

Gayle, a secretary with MS, is completely open about her illness. In fact, she routinely uses an electric scooter to get from place to place at the office. "People try to hitch rides," she jokes. Kevin takes the opposite approach. "I've learned how to cover losing my balance," he says. "I'm not going to tell anyone I have MS because they might think I can't do my job."

Whose approach is better? Should people with MS disclose or hide their illness in the workplace? This is just one of many work-related questions facing people with multiple sclerosis. Others include:

- Will I face discrimination on the job because I have MS?

- Will my coworkers lose faith in my abilities if they know I have MS?

- Will I be passed over for a promotion?

- Will MS interfere with my job performance?

- If I interview for a new job, should I tell the employer that I have MS?

- If I'm forced to give up my job because of MS, who will support my family?

There is no one right answer to each question, and each person with MS must decide for himself or herself how to handle workplace issues. The answers will depend on the person's job demands, symptoms, and financial needs.

A few things are clear, though. On the positive side, many people with mild MS encounter few interruptions in their job routines and continue to work normally for many years after an MS diagnosis. Many experts think that working helps people with MS keep a positive attitude. "Not only can people with MS continue to work, but in most cases it's in their best interests to do so," explains Gary Sumner, a former manager with the National Multiple Sclerosis Society. "They are better off psychologically, as well as physically, if they stay on the job."

Unfortunately, the employment situation is not always so positive. Although assistance devices such as scooters, vision aids, and modified office furniture can help, fatigue, vision problems, and other symptoms might eventually make it very difficult for people with MS to stay on the job. By law (the Americans with Disabilities Act of 1990), employers cannot discriminate against people with MS or other disabilities, and large employers must try to accommodate the special needs of disabled workers. In reality, though, people with MS do face discrimination. "I wasn't technically fired," explains Danny, a violinist with a major symphony, "but gradually I was demoted, from first violinist to the back of the second violins. I was told, 'We won't need you for next month's concert.' Eventually, I ended up quitting my job, because I wasn't doing it anyway."

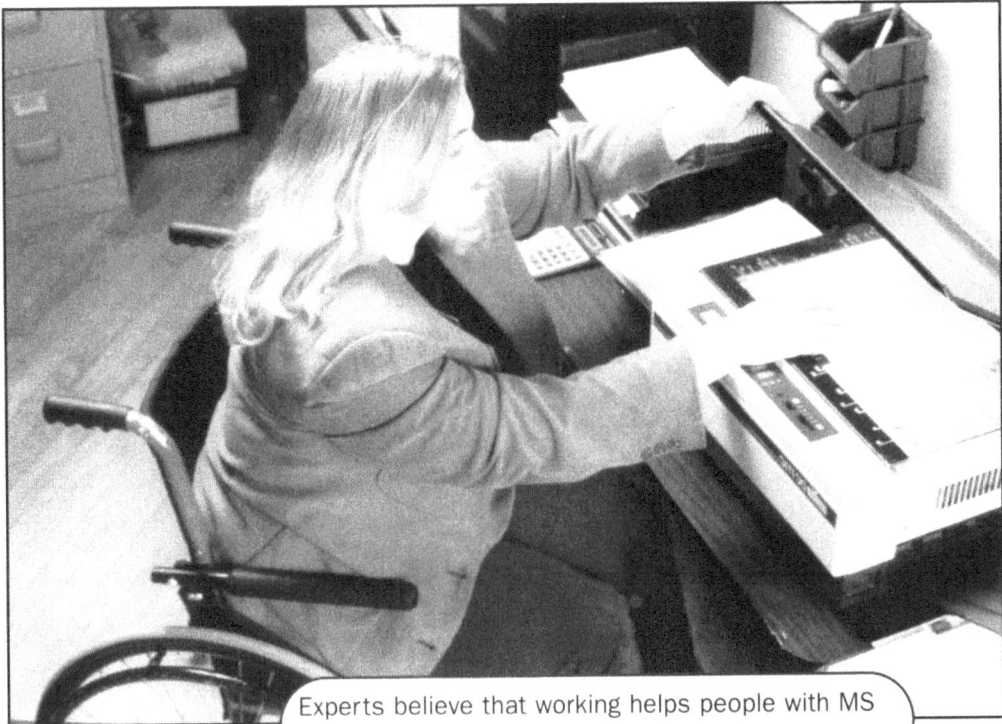

Experts believe that working helps people with MS to be independent and maintain a positive attitude.

Losing a career because of MS can be very painful. Lost income is just one negative result. Jobs often provide us with meaningful challenges, self-confidence, and a sense of satisfaction and self-worth. Losing a satisfying job, and all its benefits, can be one of the most difficult parts of dealing with multiple sclerosis.

Medical Expenses

Along with all the other obstacles, physical and emotional, MS presents many financial burdens. Medical care, physical and occupational therapy, medicines, mobility equipment, transportation, home health or nursing care, and home renovations are expensive. If a person with MS decides to quit working, his or her income will be lost.

Financial situations vary from person to person and family to family. Sometimes, a healthy partner might take a second job to cope with health care expenses or to make up for the sick partner's lost income. The family might move into cheaper housing, or the person with MS might move in with relatives for financial (and emotional) support.

Sometimes health insurance will pay for some costs associated with MS. Other times, a person with MS might qualify for Social Security Disability, a federal government assistance program. Medicare and Medicaid are federal programs that specifically cover medical bills for disabled people. Other state and federal programs provide funds for special equipment, home health care, and housing for the disabled. Renovations made to assist a disabled person at home are tax deductible. To find out what resources and funds are available, people with MS can contact government agencies and groups such as the National Multiple Sclerosis Society.

Chapter Six

Fighting Ignorance

*E*lizabeth's mom made the best cookies in the world—butterscotch raisin with chocolate chips. "Wait until you taste my mom's cookies," Elizabeth bragged to the girls in her Brownie troop before the big holiday party. All the parents were making food for the party, but Elizabeth knew that her mom was the best cook of all.

"I don't want to eat your mom's cookies," a girl named Kallie snapped back. "My dad says that your mom has AIDS." Elizabeth turned red in the face. Her mom had a disease called MS, not AIDS. And what did that have to do with anything, anyway? What did that have to do with eating the best cookies in the world?

Ignorance is one of the biggest problems that people with MS face. Those who are ignorant about MS—and other disabilities—are likely to make hurtful, inaccurate, and insensitive comments to and about people with MS. Elizabeth's friend Kallie learned some harmful lessons from her father. Not only was he ignorant about MS—and AIDS, for that matter—but he also taught his daughter to be ignorant, prejudiced, and insensitive just like himself.

Our society makes a big fuss over movie stars, runway models, teen sensations—the more glitzy and gorgeous, the better. People in wheelchairs, people with slurred speech, and people who use canes don't fit this glamorous ideal. What's more, many people are uncomfortable around those with disabilities. Perhaps they're frightened that they'll catch whatever the person has, or that they'll need to use a wheelchair themselves someday.

Whatever the reasons, people with MS encounter prejudice on a regular basis. One man says that waiters and waitresses often ask his wife, "What would your husband like to order?" They think that because his legs don't work properly, his mind must not work right either. People who slur their speech might be labeled mentally retarded, when in fact MS has affected the muscles they need to speak—not the brain power behind the words.

People with MS sometimes face a funny dilemma. Unless they use a cane, scooter, or wheelchair, they don't usually appear to be sick. Other people expect them to act just like everyone else—fit and healthy—and can't under-stand any sudden strange behavior. Carol tells a story: "Soon after I was diagnosed, but not using a cane in pub-lic yet, I knocked some jars of pickles off a shelf in a gro-cery store. The owner assumed that I was drunk and called the police." The incident left Carol feeling embar-rassed and humiliated. On other occasions, she was hassled for parking in handicapped spots because, with-out her cane, people didn't realize she had MS.

What will it take to change attitudes about MS? It will take education, sensitivity, openness to differences, and the realization that people with MS have as much to offer as everyone else. Society is quick to label people with disabilities. "I am often referred to as the violin teacher with the cane," says Danny, the musician who was forced to give up his symphony job. "I hope that eventually people will look at my disability as one of my attributes, rather than as a shortcoming."

The National Multiple Sclerosis Society

One of the leaders in the fight to educate people about MS—and to end ignorance and discrimination—is the National Multiple Sclerosis Society (NMSS). The group's primary mission, though, is "to end the devas-tating effects of MS."

Through its headquarters in New York and a network of fifty state chapters, the society funds research on MS, provides education, and offers counseling, support groups, referrals, medical information, and other programs. The society also acts as an advocate for people with MS and other disabilities. Programs include:

- Physician referrals
- Assistance referrals
- Peer counseling
- Phone counseling
- Workplace advocacy
- Employment programs
- Exercise programs
- Equipment loans
- Volunteer assistance
- Education for families, caregivers, and volunteers
- Workshops and conferences for medical personnel
- Newsletters, fact sheets, and *Inside MS* magazine
- Programs for children of people with MS
- An Internet Web site [*www.nmss.org*]

The society offers its programs for free, or for a very small fee, to people with MS and their families. It uses the services of more than a million volunteers nation-wide. Fund-raising programs include the MS Bike Tour and MS Walk. Since its founding more than fifty years ago, the NMSS has invested more than $221 million into research on multiple sclerosis. This research has led to more effective diagnostic and treatment programs and will hopefully one day lead to a cure.

Until a cure is discovered, however, people with MS face an uphill battle. But they don't have to fight that battle alone. With the support of the NMSS, family, friends, and skilled professionals, people with MS are living full and meaningful lives. MS might limit them, but it doesn't shut them down. As Jimmie Heuga, 1964 Olympic bronze medalist in skiing, proclaims, "I have MS, but it doesn't have me."

Glossary

ambulatory Able to walk.

autoimmune response When the immune system, the system that normally defends the body, attacks the body's own tissue.

central nervous system The brain and spinal cord.

cognitive function The ability to think or reason.

demyelination Destruction of the myelin sheath.

evoked potentials Tests that detect a slowing down of messages in the brain.

exacerbations Times when MS symptoms flare up or grow worse; also called relapses.

genetics The study of heredity, or the way in which traits are passed from one generation to the next.

MRI (magnetic resonance imaging) Technique used to create an image of the brain or other part of the body using radio waves and a magnet.

myelin sheath   A protective covering that protects the nerves of the brain and spinal cord.

neurology   The study of the body's nervous system.

occupational therapy   Exercises and devices designed to help injured or disabled people perform day-to-day tasks more easily.

physical therapy   Treatment designed to improve strength, flexibility, and function in people who are injured or disabled.

primary-progressive MS   Multiple sclerosis that is progressive from the start, meaning that symptoms begin to worsen right away.

relapsing-remitting MS   Multiple sclerosis that is marked by relapses (exacerbations or flare-ups), followed by periods of remission (recovery).

remission   A period of recovery, when symptoms of MS lessen or do not occur at all.

sclerosis   Scarring on the myelin sheath.

secondary-progressive MS   Multiple sclerosis that begins with only mild symptoms and grows progressively worse over time.

Where to Go for Help

In the United States

Multiple Sclerosis Association of America
706 Haddonfield Road
Cherry Hill, NJ 08002
(800) LEARN MS (532-7667)
e-mail: msaa@msaa.com
Web site: http://www.msaa.com

Multiple Sclerosis Foundation
6350 N. Andrews Avenue
Fort Lauderdale, FL 33309
(800) 441-7055
e-mail: support@msfacts.org
Web site: http://www.msfacts.org

National Multiple Sclerosis Society
733 Third Avenue

New York, NY 10017
(800) FIGHT MS (344-4867)
e-mail: info@nmss.org
Web site: http://www.nmss.org

In Canada

Multiple Sclerosis Society of Canada
250 Bloor Street East, Suite 1000
Toronto, ON M4W 3P9
(416) 922-6065
e-mail: info@mssoc.ca
Web site: http://www.mssoc.ca

Self-Help Resource Center of Greater Toronto
40 Orchard Boulevard, Suite 219
Toronto, ON M4R 1B9
(888) 283-8806
e-mail: shrc@selfhelp.on.ca
Web site: http://www.selfhelp.on.ca

Web Sites

Consortium of Multiple Sclerosis Centers
http://www.mscare.org

Doctors' Guide to the Internet—Multiple Sclerosis
http://www.pslgroup.com/ms.htm

For Further Reading

Aaseng, Nathan. *Multiple Sclerosis*. New York: Franklin Watts, 2000.

Gold, Susan Dudley, and Richard Sullivan. *Multiple Sclerosis*. Parsippany, NJ: Crestwood House, 1997.

Kraft, George H. *Living with Multiple Sclerosis: A Wellness Approach*. New York: Demos Medical Publishing, 2000.

O'Conner, Paul. *Multiple Sclerosis: The Facts You Need*. Buffalo, NY: Firefly Books, 1999.

Snyder, Ron. *One Man's Battle with MS*. South Moorehead, MN: Saga Publishing, 1995.

Susman, Edward. *Multiple Sclerosis*. Springfield, NJ: Enslow, 1999.

Swank, Roy L. and Barbara Dugan. *The Multiple Sclerosis Diet Book*. New York: Doubleday, 1987.

Index

About the Author

Margaret J. Goldstein is a freelance writer. She lives in Santa Fe, New Mexico.

Photo Credits

Cover, pp. 37, and 46 © Darren Turner; p. 2 © Index Stock Imagery; p. 11 © Everett Collection; p. 21 © Steve Skjold Photographs; pp. 24, 31, and 32 © Superstock; p. 29 © CORBIS; p. 41 © Telegraph Colour Library/FPG; p. 48 © Pete Saoutos/Custom Medical Stock Photo; pp. 17 and 51 © Custom Medical Stock Photo.

www.ingramcontent.com/pod-product-compliance
Lightning Source LLC
Chambersburg PA
CBHW050910210326
41597CB00002B/82